Sous Vide Cookbook for Busy People

Learn Modern Cooking techniques to save time and money. 60 Smart Recipes for Busy People that want to cook like a pro in a few steps

Frank Kimmons

Sous Vide Cookbook for Busy People

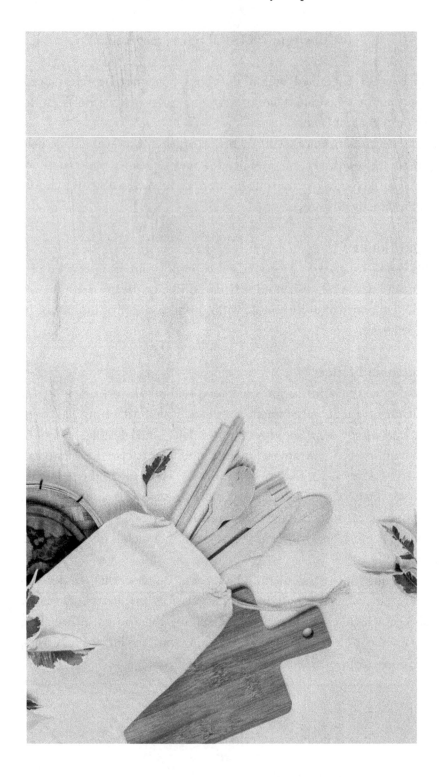

Table of Contents

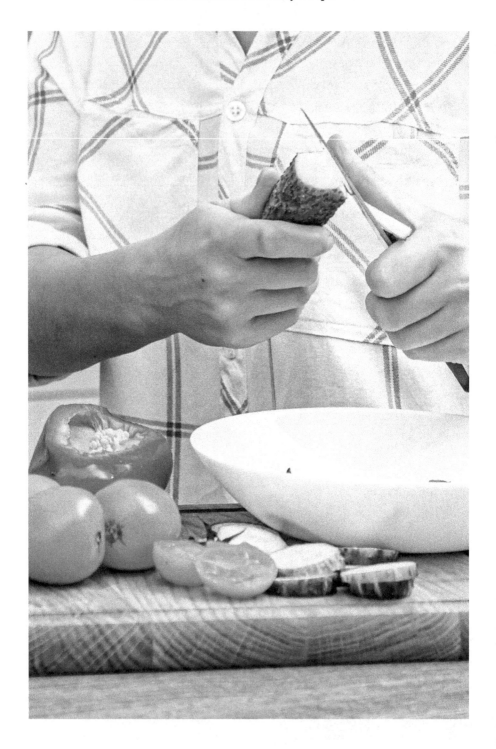

CHAPTER 1.   Red Meats

1. Chuck Shoulder with Mushrooms

Cook Time: 6 hours 15 minutes | Servings: 3

Ingredients

- 1 pound beef chuck shoulder
- 1 medium-sized carrot, sliced
- 1 large onion, chopped
- ¾ cup button mushrooms, sliced
- 1 cup beef stock
- 2 tbsp olive oil
- 4 garlic cloves, finely chopped
- Salt and black pepper to taste

Directions

Prepare a water bath and place the Sous Vide in it. Set to 136 F. Place beef chuck shoulder in a large vacuum-sealable bag along with sliced carrot, and half of the broth. Submerge the sealed bag in the water bath and cook for 6 hours. Once the timer has stopped, remove the meat from bag and pat dry.

In a pot, heat the olive oil and put in onion and garlic. Stir-fry until translucent, for 3-4 minutes. Add beef shoulder, the remaining broth, 2 cups of water, mushrooms, salt, and pepper. Bring it to a boil and reduce the heat to a minimum. Cook for an additional 5 minutes, stirring constantly.

2. Honey-Dijon Brisket

Prep + Cook Time: 48 hours 20 minutes | Servings: 12

Ingredients

- 6 pounds beef brisket
- 2 tbsp olive oil
- 4 large shallots, sliced
- 4 garlic cloves, peeled and smashed
- ¼ cup apple cider vinegar
- ½ cup tomato paste
- ½ cup honey
- ¼ cup Dijon mustard
- 2 cups water
- 1 tbsp whole black peppercorns
- 2 dried allspice berries
- Salt to taste

Directions

Prepare a water bath and place the Sous Vide in it. Set to 155 F. Heat the olive oil in a skillet over high heat and sear the brisket until golden brown on both sides. Set aside. In the same skillet on medium heat, sauté shallots and garlic for 10 minutes.

Combine vinegar, honey, tomato paste, mustard, peppercorn, water, allspice, and cloves. Add in the shallot mixture. Mix well. Place the brisket and the mixture in a vacuum-sealable bag. Release air by the water displacement method, seal, and submerge the bag in the water bath. Cook for 48 hours.

Once the timer has stopped, remove the bag and pat the meat dry. Pour the cooking juices in a saucepan over high heat and cook until the sauce has reduced by half, 10 minutes. Serve with the brisket.

3. Classic Beef Stew

Prep + Cook Time: 3 hours 15 minutes | Servings: 4

Ingredients

- 1 pound beef neck, chopped into bite-sized pieces
- ½ large eggplant, sliced
- 1 cup fire-roasted tomatoes
- 1 cup beef broth
- ½ cup burgundy
- ¼ cup vegetable oil
- 5 peppercorns, whole
- 2 tbsp butter, unsalted
- 1 bay leaf, whole
- 1 tbsp tomato paste
- ½ tbsp cayenne pepper
- ¼ tsp chili pepper (optional)
- 1 tsp salt
- Fresh parsley to garnish

Directions

Prepare a water bath and place the Sous Vide in it. Set to 135 F.

Rinse the meat under cold running water. Pat dry with kitchen paper and place on a clean working surface. Using a sharp knife, cut into bite-sized pieces.

In a large bowl, combine burgundy with oil, peppercorns, bay leaf, cayenne pepper, chili pepper, and salt. Dip meat in this mixture and refrigerate for 2 hours. Remove the meat from the marinade and pat dry with kitchen paper. Reserve the liquid. Place in a large vacuumsealable bag. Seal the bag.

Submerge the sealed bag in the water bath and cook for 1 hour. Remove from the water bath, discard the bay leaf, and transfer to a deep, heavy-bottomed pot. Add butter and gently melt over medium heat. Put in eggplants, tomatoes, and ¼ cup of the marinade. Cook for a further 5 minutes, stirring constantly. Taste, adjust the seasonings and serve garnished with chopped fresh parsley.

4. Red Wine Beef Ribs

Prep + Cook Time: 6 hours 15 minutes | Servings: 3

Ingredients

- 1 pound beef short ribs
- ¼ cup red wine
- 1 tsp honey
- ½ cup tomato paste
- 2 tbsp olive oil
- ½ cup beef stock
- ¼ cup apple cider vinegar
- 1 garlic clove, minced
- 1 tsp Paprika
- Salt and black pepper to taste

Directions

Prepare a water bath and place the Sous Vide in it. Set to 140 F. Rinse and drain the ribs. Season with salt, pepper, and paprika. Place in a vacuum-sealable bag in a single layer along with wine, tomato paste, beef broth, honey, and apple cider. Release air by the water displacement method, seal, and submerge the bag in the water bath.

Set the timer for 6 hours. Pat the ribs dry. Discard cooking liquids. In a large skillet, heat the olive oil over medium heat. Add garlic and stir-fry until translucent. Put in ribs and brown for 5 minutes per side.

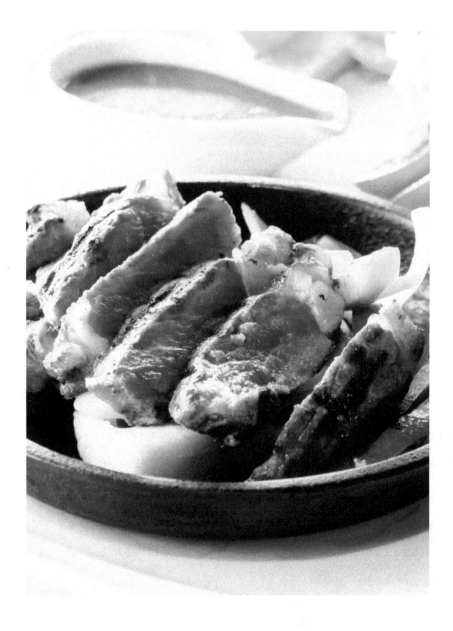

5. Beef Pepper Meat

Prep + Cook Time: 6 hours 10 minutes | Servings: 2

Ingredients

- 1 pound beef tenderloin, cut into bite-sized pieces
- 1 large onion finely chopped
- 1 tbsp butter, melted
- 1 tbsp fresh parsley, finely chopped
- 1 tsp dried thyme, ground
- 1 tbsp lemon juice, freshly squeezed
- 1 tbsp tomato paste
- Salt and black pepper to taste

Directions

Prepare a water bath and place the Sous Vide in it. Set to 158 F. Thoroughly combine all the ingredients, except for the parsley, in a large vacuum-sealable bag. Release air by the water displacement method and seal.

Submerge the bag in the water bath. Set the timer for 6 hours. Once the timer has stopped, remove from the water bath and open the bag.

Serve immediately garnished with chopped fresh parsley.

6. Stroganoff

Cook Time: 24 hours 15 minutes | Servings: 4

Ingredients

- 1 pound chuck roast, cut into chunks
- ½ onion, chopped
- 1 pound mushrooms, sliced
- 1 garlic cloves, minced
- ¼ cup white wine
- 4 tbsp Greek yogurt
- ½ cup beef stock
- 1 tbsp butter
- 1 sprig of fresh flat-leaf parsley
- Salt and black pepper to taste

Directions

Prepare a water bath and place the Sous Vide in it. Set to 140 F. Season the beef with salt and pepper. Place in a vacuum-sealable bag and seal. Immerse in the preheated water and cook for 24 hours.

The next day, melt the butter in a pan over medium heat. Put in onions and garlic and sauté until softened, about 3 minutes. Add in mushrooms and cook for an additional 5 minutes. Pour in wine and stock and cook until the mixture is reduced by half. Stir in the beef and cook for another minute. Taste and adjust the seasonings. Serve warm with minced fresh parsley.

7. Garlic Burgers

Prep + Cook Time: 70 minutes | Servings: 4

Ingredients

- 1 pound lean ground beef
- 3 garlic cloves, crushed
- 2 tbsp breadcrumbs
- 3 eggs, beaten
- 4 burger buns
- 4 crisphead lettuce leaves
- 4 tomato slices
- ¼ cup lentils, soaked
- ¼ cup oil, divided in half
- 1 tbsp cilantro, finely chopped
- Salt and black pepper to taste

Directions

Prepare a water bath, place Sous Vide in it, and set to 139 F. Meanwhile, in a bowl, combine lentils with beef, garlic, cilantro, breadcrumbs, eggs, and three tablespoons of oil. Season with salt and black pepper. Using your hands, shape burgers and lay on a lightly floured working surface. Place each burger in a vacuum-sealable bag and seal. Submerge in the water bath and cook for 1 hour.

Once the timer has stopped, remove the burgers from the bag and pat them dry with paper towel. Set aside. Heat the remaining oil in a large skillet. Brown burgers for 2-3 minutes on each side for extra crispiness. Drizzle burgers with your favorite sauce and transfer to buns. Garnish as with lettuce and tomato and serve immediately.

8. Fillet with Baby Carrots

Cook Time: 2 hours 15 minutes | Servings: 5

Ingredients

- 2 pounds beef fillet
- 7 baby carrots, sliced
- onion, chopped
- 1 cup tomato paste
- 2 tbsp vegetable oil
- tbsp fresh parsley, finely chopped
- Salt and black pepper to taste

Directions

Prepare a water bath and place the Sous Vide in it. Set to 133 F. Wash and pat dry the meat with kitchen paper. Using a sharp knife, cut into bite-sized pieces and season with salt and pepper. In a skillet, brown beef in oil over medium heat, turning to brown equally for 5 minutes. Add the carrots and onion and cook until softened, about 2 minutes. Stir in tomato paste, salt, and pepper. Pour in ½ cup of water.

Remove from the heat and transfer to a large vacuum-sealable bag in a single layer. Release air by the water displacement method, seal, and submerge the bag in the water bath. Set the timer for 2 hours. Remove the bag from the bath and transfer contents to serving plate.

Serve garnished with fresh parsley.

9. Ground Beef Stew

Prep + Cook Time: 60 minutes | Servings: 3

Ingredients

- 4 medium-sized eggplants, halved
- ½ cup lean ground beef
- 2 medium-size tomatoes, chopped
- ¼ cup extra virgin olive oil
- 2 tbsp toasted almonds, finely chopped
- 1 tbsp fresh celery leaves, chopped
- Salt and black pepper to taste
- 1 tsp thyme

Directions

Prepare a water bath and place the Sous Vide in it. Set to 180 F. Slice eggplants in half, lengthwise. Scoop the flesh and transfer to a bowl. Generously sprinkle with salt and let sit for ten minutes. Heat 3 tablespoons of oil over medium heat. Briefly fry the eggplants, for 3 minutes on each side and remove from the frying pan. Use some kitchen paper to soak up the excess oil. Set aside.

Put the ground beef in the same frying pan. Stir-fry for 5 minutes, stir in tomatoes and simmer until the tomatoes have softened. Add in eggplants, almonds and celery leaves and cook for 5 minutes. Turn off heat and stir in thyme. Transfer everything to a large vacuum-sealable bag. Release air by the water displacement method, seal, and submerge the bag in the water bath. Set the timer for 40 minutes.

Once the timer has stopped, remove the bag and pour the contents over a large bowl. Taste and adjust the seasonings. Serve garnished with parsley, if desired.

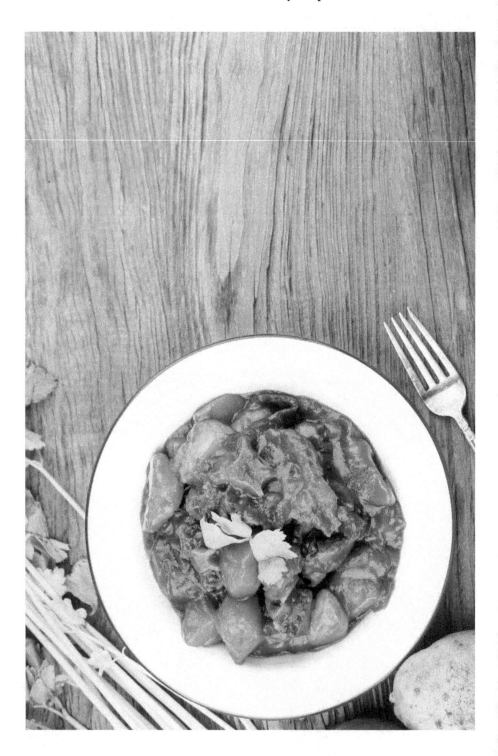

CHAPTER 2.   Pork

10.Tomato Pork Chops with Potato Puree

Prep + Cook Time: 5 hours 40 minutes | Servings: 4

Ingredients

- 1 pound skinless pork chops
- Salt and black pepper to taste
- 1 cup beef stock
- ½ cup tomato sauce
- 1 stalk celery, cut up into 1-inch dice
- 1 quartered shallot
- 3 sprigs fresh thyme
- 1 oz red mashed potatoes

Directions

Prepare a water bath and place the Sous Vide in it. Set to 182 F. Sprinkle the chops with salt and pepper, then place in a vacuumsealable bag. Add in stock, tomato sauce, shallot, whiskey, celery, and thyme. Release air by the water displacement method, seal, and submerge the bag in the water bath. Cook for 5 hours.

Once the timer has stopped, remove the chops and transfer to a plate. Reserve the cooking liquids. Heat a saucepan over high heat and pour the drained juices; let simmer.

Reduce the heat and stir for 20 minutes. Then add in chops and cook for 2-3 more minutes. Serve with potato puree.

11. Rosemary Pork Tenderloin

Prep + Cook Time: 2 hours 15 minutes | Servings: 4

Ingredients

- 1 pound pork tenderloin
- 2 garlic cloves
- 2 sprigs rosemary
- 1 tbsp dried rosemary
- Salt and black pepper to taste
- 1 tbsp olive oil

Directions

Prepare a water bath and place the Sous Vide in it. Set to 140 F. Season the meat with salt, rosemary and pepper and place in a vacuum-sealable bag with the garlic and rosemary spring inside. Release air by the water displacement method, seal, and submerge the bag in the water bath. Set the timer for 2 hours. Once the timer has stopped, remove the bag. Heat oil in a pan over medium heat.

Sear the meat on all sides for about 2 minutes.

12.Paprika Tenderloin with Herbs

Prep + Cook Time: 2 hours 20 minutes | Servings: 4

Ingredients

- 1 pound pork tenderloin, trimmed
- Salt and black pepper to taste
- 1 tbsp chopped fresh basil
- tbsp chopped fresh parsley
- 1 tablespoon paprika
- 2 tbsp butter, melted

Directions

Prepare a water bath and place the Sous Vide in it. Set to 134 F. Combine the basil, paprika, and parsley. Rub the tenderloin with salt, pepper, and herb mixture. Place in a vacuum-sealable bag. Add in 1 tbsp of butter. Release air by the water displacement method, seal, and submerge the bag in the water bath. Cook for 2 hours.

Once done, remove the tenderloin and transfer to a heated with the remaining butter skillet. Sear the for 1-2 minutes on each side. Remove and allow resting for 5 minutes. Cut the tenderloin into medallions. Serve.

13.Paprika Pancetta with Pearl Onions

Prep + Cook Time: 1 hour 50 minutes | Servings: 4

Ingredients

- 1 pound pearl onions, peeled

- 4 pancetta slices, crumbled and cooked

- 1 tbsp thyme

- 1 tsp paprika

Directions

Prepare a water bath and place Sous Vide in it. Set to 186 F. Place pancetta, pearl onions, thyme, and paprika in a vacuum-sealable bag. Release air by the water displacement method, seal and submerge the bag in the bath. Cook for 90 minutes. Once done, remove the bag and discard the cooking juices.

14. Toasts with Eggs & Crispy Pancetta

Prep + Cook Time: 70 minutes | Servings: 2

Ingredients

- 4 large egg yolks
- 2 slices pancetta
- 4 slices toasted bread

Directions

Prepare a water bath and place the Sous Vide in it. Set to 143 F. Place the egg yolks in a vacuum-sealable bag. Release air by the water displacement method, seal, and submerge the bag in the water bath. Cook for 60 minutes.

Meanwhile, cut the pancetta in slices and fry until crisp.

Transfer to a baking sheet. Once the timer has stopped, remove the yolks and place them over the toasted bread. Top with pancetta and serve.

CHAPTER 3.   Poultry

15.Paprika Chicken Lunch

Prep + Cook Time: 1 hour 15 minutes | Servings: 2

Ingredients

- 1 boneless chicken breast, halved
- Salt and black pepper to taste
- Pepper to taste
- 1 tbsp paprika
- 1 tbsp garlic powder

Directions

Prepare a water bath and place the Sous Vide in it. Set to 149 F. Drain the chicken and pat dry with a baking sheet. Season with garlic powder, paprika, pepper, and salt. Place in a vacuum-sealable bag. Release air by the water displacement method, seal and submerge in the water bath. Cook for 1 hour. Once the timer has stopped, remove the chicken and serve.

16. Breasts with Harissa Sauce

Time: 65 minutes | Servings: 4

Ingredients

- pound chicken breasts, cubed
- 1stalk of fresh lemongrass, chopped
- 2 tbsp fish sauce
- tbsp coconut sugar
- Salt to taste
- tbsp harissa sauce

Directions

Prepare a water bath and place the Sous Vide in it. Set to 149 F. In a blender, pulse lemongrass, fish sauce, sugar, and salt. Marinade the chicken with the sauce and make brochettes.

Place it in a vacuumsealable bag. Release air by the water displacement method, seal, and submerge the bag in the water bath. Cook for 45 minutes.

Once the timer has stopped, remove the bag and transfer to a cold water bath. Remove the chicken and whisk with harissa sauce. Heat a skillet over medium heat and sear the chicken. Serve.

17.Garlic Chicken with Mushrooms

Prep + Cook Time: 2 hours 15 minutes | Servings: 6

Ingredients

- 2 pounds chicken thighs, skinless
- 1 pound cremini mushrooms, sliced
- 1 cup chicken stock
- 1 garlic clove, crushed
- 4 tbsp olive oil
- ½ tsp onion powder
- ½ tsp sage leaves, dried
- ¼ tsp cayenne pepper
- Salt and black pepper to taste

Directions

Wash the thighs thoroughly under cold running water. Pat dry with kitchen paper and set aside. In a large skillet, heat the olive oil over medium heat. Brown both sides of the chicken thighs for 2 minutes. Set aside. Add garlic to the skillet and sauté until lightly brown. Stir in mushrooms, pour in stock, and cook until it reaches to a boil. Remove and set aside. Season the thighs with salt, pepper, cayenne pepper, and onion powder. Place in a large vacuum-sealable bag along with mushrooms and sage. Seal the bag and cook en Sous Vide for 2 hours at 149 F.

18. Thighs with Herbs

Time: 4 hours 10 minutes | Servings: 4

Ingredients

- 1 pound chicken thighs
- 1 cup extra virgin olive oil
- ¼ cup apple cider vinegar
- 3 garlic cloves, crushed
- ½ cup freshly squeezed lemon juice
- 1 tbsp fresh basil, chopped
- 2 tbsp fresh thyme, chopped
- 1 tbsp fresh rosemary, chopped
- 1 tsp cayenne pepper
- 1 tsp salt

Directions

Rinse the meat under cold running water and place in a large colander to drain. Set aside. In a large bowl, combine olive oil with apple cider vinegar, garlic, lemon juice, basil, thyme, rosemary, salt, and cayenne pepper. Submerge thighs into this mixture and refrigerate for one hour. Remove the meat from the marinade and drain. Place in a large vacuum-sealable bag and cook en Sous Vide for 3 hours at 149 F.

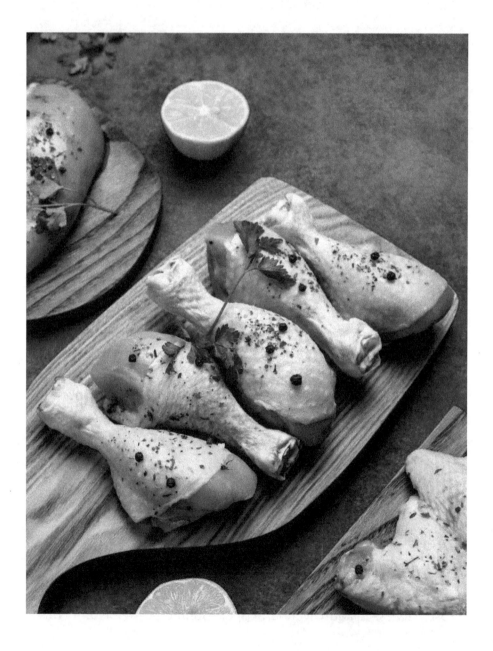

19.Almond Butternut Squash & Chicken Salad

Prep + Cook Time: 1 hour 15 minutes | Servings: 2

Ingredients

- 4 cups butternut squash, cubed and roasted
- 6 chicken tenderloins
- 4 cups rocket tomatoes
- 4 tbsp sliced almonds
- Juice of 1 lemon
- 2 tbsp olive oil
- 4 tbsp red onion, chopped
- 1 tbsp paprika
- 1 tbsp turmeric
- 1 tbsp cumin Salt to taste

Directions

Prepare a water bath and place the Sous Vide in it. Set to 138 F. Place the chicken and all the spices in a vacuum-sealable bag. Shake well. Release air by the water displacement method, seal, and submerge the bag in the water bath. Cook for 60 minutes. Once the timer has stopped, remove the chic and transfer to a heated skillet. Sear for 1 minute on each side. In a bowl, combine the remaining ingredients. Serve with chicken on top.

20.   Pudding with Artichoke Hearts

Time: 1 hour and 30 minutes | Servings: 3

Ingredients

- 1 pound chicken breasts
- 2 medium-sized artichokes
- 2 tbsp butter
- 2 tbsp extra virgin olive oil
- 1 lemon, juiced
- 2 tsp fresh parsley, finely chopped
- Salt and black pepper to taste
- ½ tsp chili pepper

Directions

Thoroughly rinse the meat and pat dry with kitchen paper. Using a sharp paring knife, cut the meat into smaller pieces and remove the bones. Rub with olive oil and set aside.

Heat the sauté pan over medium heat. Turn the heat down slightly to medium and add in the meat. Cook for 3 minutes until golden on both sides. Remove from the heat and transfer to a large vacuum-sealable bag. Seal the bag and cook en Sous Vide for one hour at 149 F.

Meanwhile, prepare the artichoke. Cut the lemon onto halves and squeeze the juice into a small bowl. Divide the juice in half and set aside. Using a sharp paring knife, trim off the outer leaves until you reach the yellow and soft ones. Trim off the green outer skin around the artichoke base and steam. Make sure to remove the 'hairs' around the artichoke heart. They are inedible so simply throw them away.

Cut artichoke into half-inch pieces. Rub with half of lemon juice and place in a heavy-bottomed pot. Add enough water to cover and cook until completely fork-tender. Remove from the heat and drain. Chill for a while at room temperature. Cut each piece into thin strips.

Now combine artichoke with chicken meat in a large bowl. Stir in salt, pepper, and the remaining lemon juice. Melt butter over medium heat and drizzle over pudding. Sprinkle with chili pepper and serve.

21. Cilantro Chicken with Peanut Butter Sauce

Prep + Cook Time: 1 hour 40 minutes | Servings: 2

Ingredients

- 4 chicken breasts
- bag mixed salad
- 1 bunch cilantro
- 2 cucumbers
- carrots
- 1 pack wonton wrappers
- 2 tbsp vegetable oil
- ¼ cup peanut butter
- Juice of 1 lime
- 2 tbsp chopped cilantro
- 3 cloves garlic
- tbsp fresh ginger
- ½ cup water
- 2 tbsp white vinegar
- tbsp soy sauce
- tsp fish sauce
- 1 tsp sesame oil
- tbsp canola oil

Directions

Prepare a water bath and place the Sous Vide in it. Set to 149 F. Season the chicken with salt and pepper and place in a vacuumsealable bag. Release air by the water displacement method, seal, and submerge the bag in the water bath. Cook for 60 minutes. Chop the cucumber, cilantro and carrots and combine with the salad. Heat the oil in a pot over medium heat. Slice the wonton wrappers in pieces and fry until crispy.

In a food processor, put peanut butter, lime juice, fresh ginger, cilantro, water, white vinegar, fish sauce, soy sauce, sesame, and canola oil. Blend until smooth. Once the timer ends, remove the chicken and transfer to a hot skillet. Sear for 30 seconds per side. Mix the wonton strips with the salad. Slice the chicken. Serve on top of the salad. Drizzle with the dressing.

22.   Chicken & Walnut Salad

Prep + Cook Time: 2 hours 20 minutes | Servings: 4

Ingredients

- 2 skinless chicken breasts, boneless
- Salt and black pepper to taste
- 1 tbsp corn oil
- 1 apple, cored and diced
- 1 tsp lime juice
- ½ cup white grapes, cut in half
- 1 stick rib celery, diced
- 1/3 cup mayonnaise
- 2 tsp Chardonnay wine
- 1 tsp Dijon mustard
- 1 head Romaine lettuce
- ½ cup walnuts, toasted and chopped

Directions

Prepare a water bath and place the Sous Vide in it. Set to 146 F. Place the chicken in a vacuum-sealable bag and season with salt and pepper. Release air by the water displacement method, seal, and submerge the bag in the water bath. Cook for 2 hours. Once the timer has stopped, remove the bag and discard cooking juices. In a large bowl, toss apple slices with lime juice. Add in celery and white grapes. Mix well.

In another bowl, stir the mayonnaise, Dijon mustard and Chardonnay wine. Pour the mixture over the fruit and mix well. Chop the chicken and put in a medium bowl, season with salt and combine well. Put the chicken in the salad bowl. Colocate the romaine lettuce in salad bowls and place salad on top. Garnish with walnuts.

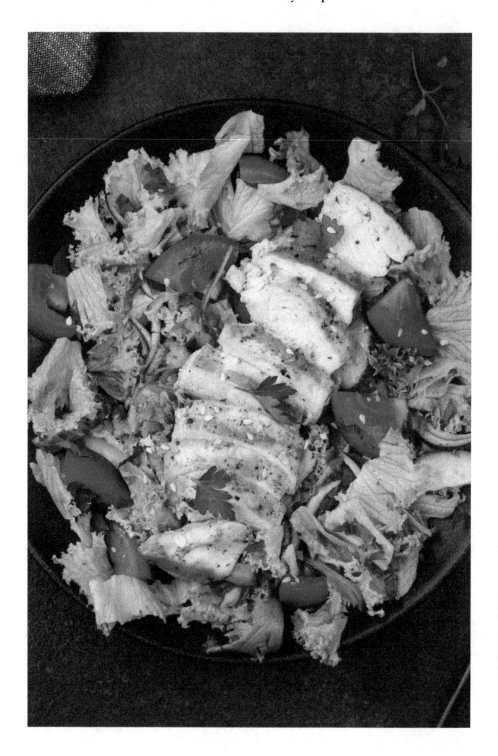

CHAPTER 4.   Fish & Seafood

23.   Savory Creamy Cod with Parsley

Prep + Cook Time: 40 minutes | Servings: 6

Ingredients

For Cod

- 6 cod fillets
- Salt to taste
- 1 tbsp olive oil
- 3 sprigs fresh parsley
- For Sauce
- 1 cup white wine
- cup half-and-half cream
- 1 finely chopped white onion
- 2 tbsp dill, chopped
- tsp black peppercorns

Directions

Prepare a water bath and place the Sous Vide in it. Set to 148 F.
Place seasoned with salt cod fillets in vacuum-sealable bags. Add
olive oil and parsley. Release air by the water displacement

method, seal, and submerge the bag in the water bath. Cook for 30 minutes.

Heat a saucepan over medium heat, add in wine, onion, black peppercorns and cook until reduced. Stir in half-and-half cream until thickened. Once the timer has stopped, plate the fish and drizzle with sauce.

24.   Thai Salmon with Cauliflower & Egg Noodles

Prep + Cook Time: 55 minutes | Servings: 2

Ingredients

- 2 skin-on salmon fillets
- Salt and black pepper to taste
- 1 tbsp olive oil
- 4 ½ tbsp soy sauce
- 2 tbsp minced fresh ginger
- 2 thinly sliced Thai Chilis
- 6 tbsp sesame oil
- 4 oz prepared egg noodles
- 6 oz cooked cauliflower florets
- 5 tsp sesame seeds

Directions

Prepare a water bath and place the Sous Vide in it. Set to 149 F. Prepare a baking tray lined with aluminium foil and put the salmon, season with salt and pepper and cover with another aluminium sheet. Bake in the oven for 30 minutes. Remove the baked salmon to a vacuum-sealable bag. Release air by the water displacement method, seal, and submerge the bag in the water bath. Cook for 8 minutes.

In a bowl, mix ginger, chilis, 4 tbsp of soy sauce, and 4 tbsp of sesame oil. Once the timer has stopped, remove the bag and transfer the salmon to a noodle bowl. Garnish with toasted seeds and salmon skin. Sprinkle with the ginger-chili sauce and serve.

25.   Basil Cod Stew

Prep + Cook Time: 50 minutes | Servings: 4

Ingredients

- 1 pound cod fillet
- 1 cup fire-roasted tomatoes
- tbsp basil, dried
- 1 cup fish stock
- 2 tbsp tomato paste
- 3 celery stalks, finely chopped
- carrot, sliced
- ¼ cup olive oil
- onion, finely chopped
- ½ cup button mushrooms

Directions

Heat olive oil in a large skillet, over medium heat. Add celery, onions, and carrot. Stir-fry for 10 minutes. Remove from the heat and transfer to a vacuum-sealable bag along with other ingredients. Cook in sous vide for 40 minutes at 122 F.

Serve and enjoy!

26.   Easy Tilapia

Prep + Cook Time: 1 hour 10 minutes | Servings: 3

Ingredients

- 3 (4 oz) tilapia fillets
- 3 tbsp butter
- 1 tbsp apple cider vinegar
- Salt and black pepper to taste

Directions

Make a water bath, place Sous Vide in it, and set to 124 F. Season the tilapia with pepper and salt and place in a vacuum-sealable bag. Release air by the water displacement method and seal the bag.

Submerge it in the water bath and set the timer for 1 hour. Once the timer has stopped, remove and unseal the bag. Put a skillet over medium heat and add butter and vinegar. Simmer and stir continually to reduce vinegar by half. Add the tilapia and sear slightly. Season with salt and pepper as desired. Serve and enjoy!

27.   Sesame-Crusted Cod Fillet

Prep + Cook Time: 45 minutes | Servings: 2

Ingredients

- 1 large cod fillet
- 2 tbsp sesame paste
- 1 ½ tbsp brown sugar
- 2 tbsp fish sauce
- 2 tbsp butter
- Sesame seeds

Directions

Prepare a water bath and place the Sous Vide in it. Set to 131 F. Soak cod with the brown sugar, sesame paste and fish sauce mixture. Place in a vacuum-sealable bag. Release air by the water displacement method, seal, and submerge the bag in the water bath. Cook for 30 minutes. Melt butter in a skillet over medium heat.

Once the timer has stopped, remove the cod and transfer to the skillet and sear for 1 minute. Serve onto a platter. Pour cooking juices into the skillet and cook until reduced. Add 1 tbsp of butter and mix. Top cod with the sauce and garnish with sesame seeds. Serve with rice.

28.   Salmon with Asparagus

Prep + Cook Time: 3 hours 15 minutes | Servings: 6

Ingredients

- 1 pound wild salmon fillet

- 1 tbsp olive oil

- 1 tbsp dried oregano

- 12 medium asparagus spears

- 4 white onion rings

- 1 tbsp fresh parsley

- Salt and black pepper to taste

Directions

Season the fillet with oregano, salt, and pepper on both sides and lightly brush with olive oil. Place in a large vacuum-sealable along with other ingredients. Combine all spices in a mixing bowl. Rub the mixture evenly on both sides of the steak and place in a large vacuum-sealable bag. Seal the bag and cook in sous vide for 3 hours at 136 F. Serve and enjoy!

29.   Creamy Salmon with Spinach &

Mustard Sauce

Prep + Cook Time: 55 minutes | Servings: 2

Ingredients

- 4 skinless salmon fillets
- 1 large bunch of spinach
- ½ cup Dijon mustard
- 1 cup heavy cream
- 1 cup half-and-half cream
- 1 tbsp lemon juice
- Salt and black pepper to taste

Directions

Prepare a water bath and place the Sous Vide in it. Set to 115 F. Place the salmon seasoned with salt in a vacuum-sealable bag. Seal and submerge the bag in the bath. Cook for 45 minutes.

Heat a pot over medium heat and cook spinach until softened. Lower the heat and pour in lemon juice, pepper and salt. Keep cooking. Heat a saucepan over medium heat and combine the half-and-half cream and Dijon mustard. Lower the heat and cook. Season with salt and pepper. Once the timer has stopped, remove the salmon and transfer to a plate. Drizzle with sauce. Serve with spinach.

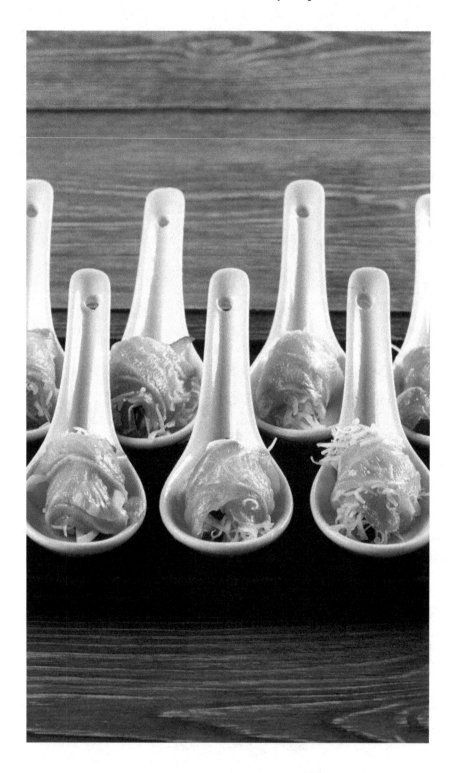

CHAPTER 5. Eggs

30. Hard-Boiled Eggs

Prep + Cook Time: 1 hour 10 minutes | Servings: 3

Ingredients

- 3 large eggs Ice bath

Directions

Make a water bath, place Sous Vide in it, and set to 165 F. Place the eggs in the water bath and set the timer for 1 hour. Once the timer has stopped, transfer the eggs to an ice bath. Peel eggs. Serve as a snack or in salads.

31. Tomato Shakshuka

Prep + Cook Time: 2 hours 10 minutes | Servings: 3

Ingredients

- 28 ounces canned crushed tomatoes
- 6 eggs - 1 tbsp paprika
- 2 garlic cloves, minced
- Salt and black pepper to taste
- 2 tsp cumin
- ¼ cup minced cilantro

Directions

Prepare a water bath and place the Sous Vide in it. Set to 148 F. Place the eggs in a vacuum-sealable bag. Release air by the water displacement method, seal, and submerge the bag in the water bath. Combine the remaining ingredients in another vacuum-sealable bag. Set the timer for 2 hours. Divide the tomato sauce between three bowls. Once the timer has stopped, remove the bag. Peel the eggs and place 2 in each bowl.

CHAPTER 6.   Appetizers and Snacks

32.   Radish Cheese Dip

Prep + Cook Time: 1 hour 15 minutes | Servings: 4

Ingredients

- 30 radishes, green leaves removed
- 1 tbsp Chardonnay vinegar
- Sugar to taste - 1 cup water for steaming
- 1 tbsp grapeseed oil 12 oz cream cheese

Directions

Make a water bath, place Sous Vide in it, and set to 183 F. Put the radishes, salt, pepper, water, sugar, and vinegar in a vacuum-sealable bag. Release air from the bag, seal and submerge in the water bath. Cook for 1 hour.   Once the timer has stopped, remove the bag, unseal and transfer the radishes with a little steaming water into a blender. Add cream cheese and puree to get a smooth paste. Serve.

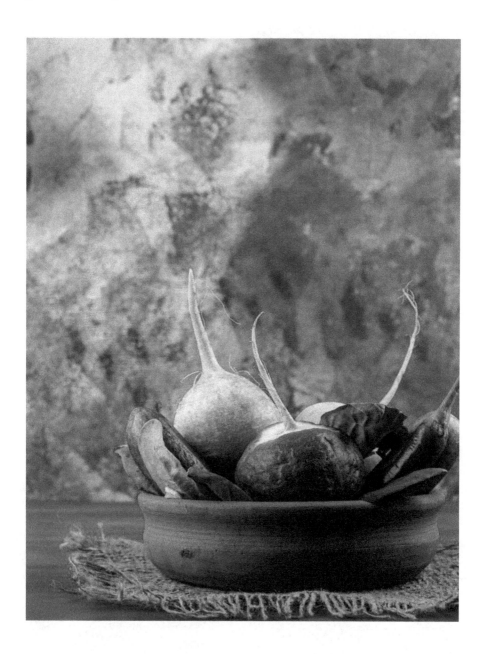

33.   Celery Dip

Prep + Cook Time: 50 minutes | Servings: 3

Ingredients

- ½ lb celery root, sliced
- 1 cup heavy cream
- 3 tbsp butter
- 1 tbsp lemon juice Salt to taste

Directions

Make a water bath, place Sous Vide in it, and set to 183 F. Place celery, heavy cream, lemon juice, butter, and salt in a vacuumsealable bag. Release air from the bag, seal and submerge in the bath. Cook for 40 minutes. Once the timer has stopped, remove and unseal the bag. Puree the ingredients using a blender. Serve.

34.   Chicken & Mushrooms in Marsala Sauce

Prep + Cook Time: 2 hours 25 minutes | Servings: 2

Ingredients

- 2 chicken breasts
- 1 cup Marsala wine
- 1 cup chicken broth
- 14 ounces mushrooms, sliced
- ½ tbsp flour
- 1 tbsp butter
- Salt and black pepper to taste
- 2 garlic cloves, minced
- 1 shallot, minced

Directions

Prepare a water bath and place the Sous Vide in it. Set to 140 F. Season the chicken with salt and pepper and place in a vacuumsealable bag along with the mushrooms. Release air by the water displacement method, seal and submerge in the water bath. Cook for 2 hours. Once the timer has stopped, remove the bag. Melt the butter in a pan over medium heat, whisk in the flour and the remaining ingredients. Cook until the sauce thickens. Add chicken and cook for 1 minute.

35.   White Wine Mussels

Prep + Cook Time: 1 hour 20 minutes | Servings: 3

Ingredients

- 1 pound fresh mussels
- 3 tbsp extra virgin olive oil
- 1 cup onions, finely chopped
- ¼ cup fresh parsley, finely chopped
- 3 tbsp fresh thyme, chopped
- 1 tbsp lemon zest
- 1 cup dry white wine

Directions

Heat the oil in a medium-sized skillet over medium heat. Add onions and stir-fry until translucent, 3 minutes. Add lemon zest, parsley, and thyme. Give it a good stir and transfer to a vacuum-sealable bag. Add mussels and one cup of dry white wine. Seal the bag and cook in Sous Vide for 40 minutes at 104 F. Serve and enjoy!

36.　　Scallops with Bacon

Prep + Cook Time: 50 minutes | Servings: 6

Ingredients

- 10 ounces scallops
- 3 ounces bacon, sliced
- ½ onion, grated
- ½ tsp white pepper
- 1 tbsp olive oil

Directions

Prepare a water bath and place the Sous Vide in it. Set to 140 F. Top the scallops with the grated onion and wrap with bacon slices. Sprinkle with white pepper and drizzle with oil. Place in a plastic bag. Release air by the water displacement method, seal, and submerge the bag in the water bath. Set the timer for 35 minutes. Once the timer has stopped, remove the bag. Serve.

37.   Chicken Liver Spread

Prep + Cook Time: 5 hours 15 minutes | Servings: 8

Ingredients

- 1pound chicken liver
- 6 eggs
- 8 ounces bacon, minced
- 2 tbsp soy sauce
- 3 ounces shallot, chopped
- 3 tbsp vinegar
- Salt and black pepper to taste
- 4 vtbsp butter
- ½ tsp paprika

Directions

Prepare a water bath and place the Sous Vide in it. Set to 156 F. Cook the bacon in a skillet over medium heat, add shallots and cook for 3 minutes. Stir in the soy sauce and vinegar. Transfer to a blender along with the remaining ingredients. Blend until smooth. Place all the ingredients in a mason jar and seal. Cook for 5 hours. Once the timer has stopped, remove the jar and serve.

38.   Spicy Pickled Beets

Prep + Cook Time: 50 minutes |

Ingredients

- 12 oz beets, sliced ½ jalapeno pepper
- 1 diced garlic clove
- 2/3 cup white vinegar
- 2/3 cup water
- 2 tbsp pickling spice

Directions

Prepare a water bath and place the Sous Vide in it. Set to 192 F. In 5 mason jars, combine jalapeño pepper, beets and garlic cloves. Heat a saucepan and boil the pickling spice, water and white vinegar. Drain and pour over the beets mixture inside the jars. Seal and submerge the jars in the water bath. Cook for 40 minutes. Once the timer has stopped, remove the jars and allow cooling. Serve.

CHAPTER 7.   Sauces, Stocks and Broths

39.   Chicken Stock

Prep + Cook Time: 12 hours 25 minutes | Servings: 4

Ingredients

- 2 lb chicken, any parts – thighs, breasts
- 2 celery sticks, chopped
- 2 white onions, chopped

Directions

Make a water bath, place Sous Vide in it, and set to 194 F. Separate all the ingredients in 2 vacuum bags, fold the top of the bags 2–3 times. Place in the water bath. Set the timer for 12 hours.

Once the timer has stopped, remove the bags and transfer the ingredients to a pot. Boil the ingredients over high heat for 10 minutes.

Turn off heat and strain. Use the stock as a soup base.

40.　　Mustard Asparagus Dressing

Prep + Cook Time: 30 minutes | Servings: 2

Ingredients

- 1 lb large asparagus, trimmed Salt and black pepper to taste
- ¼ cup olive oil
- 1 tsp Dijon mustard
- 1 tsp dill
- 1 tsp red wine vinegar
- 1 hard-boiled egg, chopped
- Fresh parsley, chopped

Directions

Prepare a water bath and place the Sous Vide in it. Set to 186 F. Peel the bottom of the stalk and place in a vacuum-sealable bag. Release air by the water displacement method, seal, and submerge the bag in the bath.

Cook for 15 minutes. Once the timer has stopped, remove the bag and transfer to an ice bath. Separate the cooking juices. In a bowl, for the vinaigrette, combine olive oil, vinegar and mustard; stir well. Season with salt and move it to a mason jar. Seal and shake until well combined. Top with parsley, egg, and the vinaigrette.

CHAPTER 8.   Vegetarian & Vegan

41. Oregano White Beans

Prep + Cook Time: 5 hours 15 minutes | Servings: 8

Ingredients

- 12 ounces white beans
- 1 cup tomato paste
- 8 ounces veggie stock
- 1 tbsp sugar
- 3 tbsp butter
- 1 cup chopped onions
- 1 bell pepper, chopped
- 1 tbsp oregano 2 tsp paprika

Directions

Prepare a water bath and place the Sous Vide in it. Set to 185 F. Combine all the ingredients in a vacuum-sealable bag. Stir to combine. Release air by the water displacement method, seal, and submerge the bag in the water bath. Set the timer for 5 hours. Once the timer has stopped, remove the bag. Serve warm.

42.   Cabbage & Pepper in Tomato Sauce

Prep + Cook Time: 4 hours 45 minutes | Servings: 6

Ingredients

- 2 pounds cabbage, sliced
- cup sliced bell pepper
- 1 cup tomato paste - 2 onions, sliced
- tbsp sugar - Salt and black pepper to taste
- tbsp cilantro
- 1 tbsp olive oil

Directions

Prepare a water bath and place the Sous Vide in it. Set to 184 F. Place the cabbage and onion in a vacuum-sealable bag and season with the spices. Add in tomato paste and stir to combine well. Release air by the water displacement method, seal, and submerge the bag in the water bath. Set the timer for 4 hours and 30 minutes. Once the timer has stopped, remove the bag.

43. Balsamic Braised Cabbage

Prep + Cook Time: 1 hour 45 minutes | Servings: 3

Ingredients

- lb red cabbage, quartered and core removed
- 1 shallot, thinly sliced
- 2 cloves garlic, thinly sliced
- ½ tbsp balsamic vinegar
- ½ tbsp unsalted butter
- Salt to taste

Directions

Make a water bath, place Sous Vide in it, and set to 185 F. Divide cabbage and remaining ingredients into 2 vacuum-sealable bags. Release air by the water displacement method and seal the bags. Submerge them in the water bath and set the timer to cook for 1 hour 30 minutes.

Once the timer has stopped, remove and unseal the bags. Transfer the cabbage with juices into serving plates. Season with salt and vinegar to taste. Serve as a side dish.

44.   Grape Vegetable Mix

Prep + Cook Time 105 minutes | Servings: 9

Ingredients

- 8 sweet potatoes, sliced
- 2 red onions, sliced
- 4 ounces tomato, pureed
- 1 tsp minced garlic
- Salt and black pepper to taste
- 1 tsp grape juice

Directions

Prepare a water bath and place Sous Vide in it. Set to 183 F. Place all the ingredients with ¼ cup water in a vacuum-sealable bag.Release air by the water displacement method, seal, and submerge the bag in the water bath. Set the timer for 90 minutes. Once the timer has stopped, remove the bag. Serve warm.

45.   Vegetable Caponata

Prep + Cook Time: 2 hours 15 minutes | Servings: 4

Ingredients

- 4 canned plum tomatoes, crushed

- 2 bell peppers, sliced

- 2 zucchinis, sliced

- ½ onion, sliced

- 2 eggplants, sliced

- 6 garlic cloves, minced

- 2 tbsp olive oil

- 6 basil leaves

- Salt and black pepper to taste

Directions

Prepare a water bath and place the Sous Vide in it. Set to 185 F. Combine all of the ingredients in a vacuum-sealable bag. Release air by the water displacement method, seal, and submerge the bag in the water bath. Set the timer for 2 hours. Once the timer has stopped, transfer to a serving platter.

46.   Braised Swiss Chard with Lime

Prep + Cook Time: 25 minutes | Servings: 2

- 2 pounds Swiss chard
- 4 tbsp of extra virgin olive oil
- 2 garlic cloves, crushed
- 1 whole lime, juiced
- 2 tsps sea salt

Directions

Thoroughly rinse Swiss chard and drain in a colander. Using a sharp paring knife roughly chop and transfer to a large bowl. Stir in 4 tablespoons of olive oil, crushed garlic, lime juice, and sea salt. Transfer to a large vacuum-sealable bag and seal. Cook en sous vide for 10 minutes at 180 F.

47.   Root Veggie Mash

Prep + Cook Time: 3 hours 15 minutes | Servings: 4

Ingredients

- 2 parsnips, peeled and chopped
- 1 turnip, peeled and chopped
- 1 large sweet potatoes, peeled and chopped
- 1 tbsp butter
- Salt and black pepper to taste
- Pinch of nutmeg ¼ tsp thyme

Directions

Prepare a water bath and place Sous Vide in it. Set to 185 F. Place the veggies in a vacuum-sealable bag. Release air by the water displacement method, seal and submerge in the water bath. Cook for 3 hours. Once done, remove the bag and mash the veggies with a potato masher. Stir in the remaining ingredients.

48. Mustardy Lentil & Tomato Dish

Prep + Cook Time: 105 minutes | Servings: 8

Ingredients

- 2 cups lentils
- 1 can chopped tomatoes, undrained
- 1 cup green peas
- 3 cups veggie stock
- 3 cups water
- 1 onion, chopped
- carrot, sliced
- 1 tbsp butter
- 2 tbsp mustard
- 1 tsp red pepper flakes
- 2 tbsp lime juice
- Salt and black pepper to taste

Directions

Prepare a water bath and place Sous Vide in it. Set to 192 F. Place all the ingredients in a large vacuum-sealable bag. Release air by water displacement method, seal and submerge in bath. Cook for 90 minutes. Once the timer has stopped, remove the bag and transfer to a large bowl and stir before serving.

49.　　Buttery Summer Squash

Prep + Cook Time: 1 hour 35 minutes | Servings: 4

Ingredients

- 2 tbsp butter
- ¾ cup onion, chopped
- 1 ½ pounds summer squash, sliced
- Salt and black pepper to taste
- ½ cup whole milk
- 2 large whole eggs
- ½ cup crumbled plain potato chips

Directions

Prepare a water bath and place the Sous Vide in it. Set to 175 F. Grease a few jars. Heat a large skillet over medium heat and melt the butter. Add in onions and sauté for 7 minutes. Add the squash, season with salt and pepper and sauté for 10 minutes. Divide the mix in the jars. Allow it cool and set aside. Whisk the milk, salt and eggs in a bowl. Season with pepper. Pour the mixture over the jars, seal and submerge the jars in the water bath. Cook for 60 minutes. Once the timer has stopped, remove the jars and allow cooling for 5 minutes. Serve over potato chips.

50.　　Bell Pepper Rice Pilaf with Raisins

Prep + Cook Time: 3 hours 10 minutes | Servings: 6

Ingredients

- cups white rice
- 2 cups veggie stock
- ⅔ cup water
- 3 tbsp raisins, chopped
- 2 tbsp sour cream
- ½ cup chopped red onion
- bell pepper, chopped
- Salt and black pepper to taste
- tsp thyme

Directions

Prepare a water bath and place the Sous Vide in it. Set to 180 F. Place all the ingredients in a vacuum-sealable bag. Stir to combine well. Release air by the water displacement method, seal, and submerge the bag in the water bath. Set the timer for 3 hours. Once the timer has stopped, remove the bag. Serve warm.

CHAPTER 9.   Desserts & Drinks

51.Indian Lassi with Papaya

Prep + Cook Time: 32 hours 45 minutes | Servings: 8

Ingredients

- 3 cups milk
- 3 tbsp yogurt
- 2 pitted papaya, diced
- ¼ cup sugar
- 1 cup ice
- 1 tbsp vanilla extract
- ½ tsp salt
- Fresh mint leaves for garnish

Directions

Prepare a water bath and place the Sous Vide in it. Set to 115 F. Hot a saucepan over medium heat and hot the milk. Pour into canning jars and allow cooling. Pour in yogurt and seal. Submerge the jar in the water bath. Cook for 24 hours. Once the timer has stopped, remove the jar and transfer into an ice-water bath.

Transfer to the fridge and allow chilling for 8 hours. Blend the papaya, sugar, ice, vanilla, salt, 2 cups of milk and the yogurt mixture. Mix until smooth.

Garnish with mint leaves.

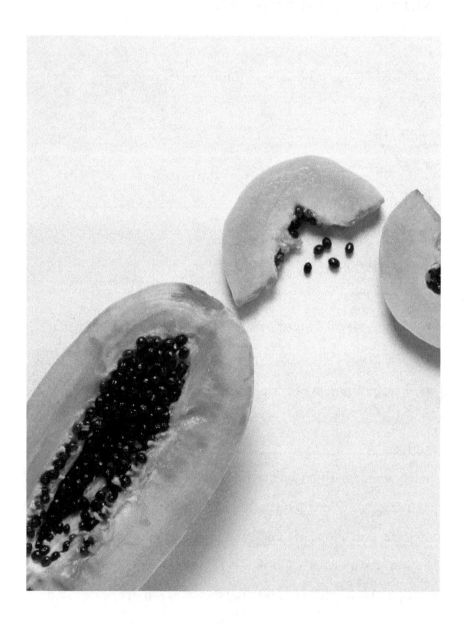

52.   Maple & Cinnamon Steel Oats

Prep + Cook Time: 3 hours 10 minutes | Servings: 2

Ingredients

- 2 cups almond milk
- ½ cup steel cut oats - ¼ tsp salt
- Cinnamon and maple syrup for topping

Directions

Prepare a water bath and place the Sous Vide in it. Set to 182 F. Combine all the ingredients, except the cinnamon and maple syrup and place in a vacuum-sealable bag. Release air by the water displacement method, seal, and submerge the bag in the water bath. Cook for 3 hours. Once the timer has stopped, remove the oats and transfer into a serving bowl. Garnish with cinnamon and maple syrup.

53.   Asian-Style Rice Pudding with Almonds

Prep + Cook Time: 7 hours 30 minutes | Servings: 5

Ingredients

- 5 tbsp basmati rice
- 2 (14-oz) cans coconut milk
- 3 tbsp sugar
- 5 cardamom pods, crushed
- 3 tbsp cashews, chopped
- Slivered almonds for garnish

Directions

Prepare a water bath and place the Sous Vide in it. Set to 182 F. In a bowl, combine the coconut milk, sugar, and 1 cup water. Pour the rice and mix well. Divide the mixture between the jars. Add a cardamom pod to each pot. Seal and submerge in the bath. Cook for 3 hours. Once the timer has stopped, remove the jars. Allow cooling for 4 hours. Serve and top with cashews and almonds.

54.   Gingered Peaches with Cardamom

Prep + Cook Time: 1 hour 15 minutes | Servings: 4

Ingredients

- 1 pound peaches, halved
- 1 tbsp butter
- 1 tsp cardamom seeds, freshly ground
- ½ tsp ground ginger
- ½ tsp salt - Fresh basil, chopped

Directions

Prepare a water bath and place the Sous Vide in it. Set to 182 F. Combine the butter, peaches, ginger, cardamom, and salt. Place in a vacuum-sealable bag. Release air by the water displacement method, seal, and submerge the bag in the water bath. Cook for 60 minutes. Once the timer has stopped, remove the bag and transfer into a bowl. Garnished with basil and serve.

55.   Maple Potato Flan

Prep + Cook Time: 1 hour 10 minutes | Servings: 6

Ingredients

- 1 cup milk
- 1 cup heavy whipping cream
- 3 whole eggs
- 3 egg yolks
- ½ cup sweet potatoes puree
- ¼ cup maple syrup
- ½ tsp pumpkin spice
- Sugar for garnish

Directions

Prepare a water bath and place Sous Vide in it. Set to 168 F. Combine the milk, heavy cream, whole eggs, egg yolks, sweet potatoes puree, maple syrup, and pumpkin spice. Mix until smooth. Pour into mason jars. Seal and submerge in the water bath. Cook for 1 hour. Once ready, remove the jars and allow chilling. Sprinkle with sugar, place under broiler until the sugar is caramelized, and serve.

56.   Homemade Vanilla Pudding

Prep + Cook Time: 55 minutes | Servings: 6

Ingredients

- 1 cup whole milk
- 1 cup whipping cream
- ½ cup sugar
- 3 large eggs (2 additional egg yolks)
- 3 tbsp cornstarch
- 1 tbsp vanilla extract
- ½ tsp salt

Directions

Prepare a water bath and place the Sous Vide in it. Set to 182 F.
In a blender, mix all the ingredients and pulse until smooth.
Transfer to a vacuum-sealable bag. Release air by the water
displacement method, seal, and submerge the bag in the water
bath. Cook for 45 minutes. Shake a few times. Once the timer
has stopped, remove the bag and transfer the contents to the
blender. Mix until smooth. Allow chilling in a bowl. Top with
strawberries.

57.　　Honey Tangerines

Prep + Cook Time: 1 hour 15 minutes | Servings: 4

Ingredients

- 1 pound tangerines
- ¼ cup honey ½ tsp salt

Directions

Prepare a water bath and place the Sous Vide in it. Set to 193 F. Slice the tangerines and remove stems and seeds. Combine the honey, tangerines and kosher salt. Place in a vacuum-sealable bag. Release air by the water displacement method, seal, and submerge the bag in the water bath. Cook for 60 minutes. Once the timer has stopped, remove the bag and cool it. Serve.

58. Coconut Banana Oatrolls with Walnuts

Prep + Cook Time: 6-10 hours 5 minutes | Servings: 4

Ingredients

- 2 cups rolled oats
- 3 cups coconut milk
- 3 cups skimmed milk
- 3 mashed bananas
- 1 tsp vanilla extract
- 1 cup of walnuts, chopped

Directions

Prepare a water bath and place the Sous Vide in it. Set to 182 F.Combine all the ingredients and place in a vacuum-sealable bag. Release air by the water displacement method, seal, and submerge the bag in the water bath. Cook for 6-10 hours. Once the timer has stopped, remove the bags and transfer the oats into serving bowls.

Top with walnuts.

59.   White Chocolate & Banana Popsicles

Prep + Cook Time: 40 minutes | Servings: 6

Ingredients

- 3 bananas - 3 tbsp peanut butter
- 3 tbsp white chocolate chips

Directions

Prepare a water bath and place the Sous Vide in it. Set to 138 F. Cut the banana in slices. Place them in a vacuum-sealable bag with white chocolate chips and peanut butter. Release air by the water displacement method, seal, and submerge the bag in the water bath. Cook for 30 minutes. Once the timer has stopped, remove the bag and transfer into popsicles molds. Allow cooling. Pop-out and serve.

60.   Citrus Piña Colada

Prep + Cook Time: 2 hours 10 minutes | Servings: 1

Ingredients

- 1 pineapple, chopped
- 3 cups white rum
- 1 tbsp coconut water
- 1 tbsp orange juice
- 1 tbsp lemon juice 1 tbsp soda water

Directions

Prepare a water bath and place the Sous Vide in it. Set to 130 F. Pour the rum and pineapple in two mason jars and seal with a lid and submerge the jars in the water bath. Cook for 2 hours.

Once the timer has stopped, remove the jars and transfer to an ice water bath. Drain the pineapple. Place into a cocktail shaker some ice, 1 ½ oz of pineapple-infused rum, coconut water, orange juice, and lemon juice. Shake for 30 seconds. Pour into a highball glass with ice.

Garnish with pineapple chunks.

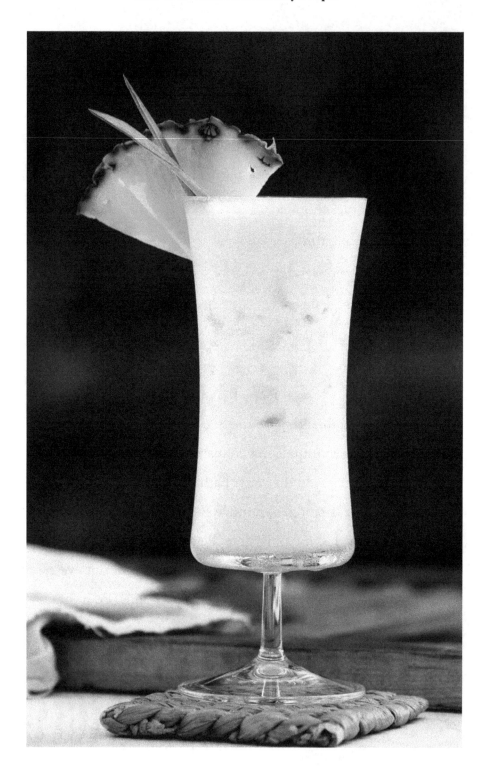

CPSIA information can be obtained
at www.ICGtesting.com
Printed in the USA
BVHW091502190521
607631BV00001B/46

9 781802 891096